DEDICATION

I dedicate this work to all those who care
so much about their holistic health!

CONTENTS

DISCLAIMER!

The information contained in this book
is for educational purposes only. The
author, Shawn Tuttle is not attempting
to prescribe a drug, diagnose, or treat
any condition, disease, or injury.

It is important that before starting any
exercise or health program, you should
receive full medical clearance from a
licensed physician.

INTRODUCTION

Except you are living on Mars, then you have probably heard about the so-called "mighty" healing powers of celery juice. You cannot scroll past three posts on Instagram without seeing a post where someone is showing a before and after picture of their body after taking celery juice.

On YouTube, celery juice videos are gathering a lot of views. On Facebook, the story is not in any way different.

Everywhere you turn to, both online and offline, the new wellness alpha and omega seems to be celery juice.

One question you might want to ask is, "*why is everybody suddenly becoming obsessed with celery juice?*" For the most part, celery has always been with us for centuries, so what is the reason for the overnight popularity it has seen these days?

Many of us have been asking these questions without getting answers. Some of us who don't want to feel left out have even jumped on the bandwagon. However, is celery juice really the "be-all end-all" that many people are touting it to be? What is in it for those who are promoting this plant as an omnipotent plant in the wellness world? Well, you will soon find out.

Sometime in mid-2018, when it seemed like the celery juice craze was at its peak, I was conversing with a friend, and somehow we started talking about the latest celery juice craze.

We are both health and fitness enthusiasts, so talking about the topic was a natural thing to do. My friend asked, "What do you think about the latest wellness fad, celery juice?" I said to him, "Once they tell you that it heals all the sicknesses in the world, rest assured, it heals nothing." I gave him that reply due to my experience drinking celery juice in the early months of 2018.

We laughed over it, but that is the ugly truth – every drug that has ever been proven to work has something specific that it heals or is known for. Unfortunately, those promoting celery juice claim that it treats all forms of sicknesses, both known and unknown. While we were still talking, my friend jokingly remarked that even the price of celery stalks had gone up significantly. He mentioned he used to buy the plant for $0.98, but the price had doubled.

I have always tried alternative medicine, and why some of them work, some others usually turn out to be a total waste of time and resources. Now, as someone who had been battling with acid reflux, which had somehow refused to go, my wife and I decided I should try celery juice, maybe for its sake. I had heard that it heals all kinds of diseases, including acid reflux, so I was enthusiastic. This was happening around January 2018.

After more than two months of drinking celery according to specifications given by Anthony William, the man who started this whole celery juice craze, it felt like I was going from bad to worse every single day.

Unlike what the other people who had tried the juice said, my case was different. Maybe, those people tried celery juice for its acclaimed ability to make the skin feel beautiful and clean; I do not know.

It could be that the juice really works to make the skin look flawless, that I cannot say. But the claim that celery juice is good for gut health is a pure lie, at least, according to my experience.

After I had tried celery juice for two months with nothing to show for it, I felt I should do some independent research and find out if the claims are valid or not. Earlier, I had read some of Anthony William's books where he maintained that celery juice was the alpha and omega.

But it was time to do independent research, and what I discovered, coupled with my experience drinking celery juice, showed that, just like the other health and fitness fads that came before it, celery juice is nothing more than a mere social media hype.

To further satisfy my curiosity about the efficacy of celery juice for the treatment of any sickness at all, I decided to use my teenage daughter as a "lab rat." As a teenage girl, she had been battling acne, so I wanted her to drink celery juice and see if anything would change. To our surprise, nothing changed after she had taken the juice on an empty stomach for more than a month.

The combined experiences of both my daughter and I show that most of the testimonials you might have seen on the internet about the healing powers of celery juice are either fake or something else gave those people the results they got.

You may ask, *"Could it mean that all the celebrities who referred to celery juice as a miracle juice were all lying in their testimonies?"* Well, I cannot state emphatically that they all lied, but we have had several instances where these celebrities lied just to promote something or an idea that one of them was pushing.

Just like the title of this book says, I have tried celery juice, so you do not have to waste both your time, energy, and money drinking it. Do not misunderstand me, please! Celery in itself is a perfectly good plant, which sure has some health benefits. However, if you want to pulverize some celery stalks because one person on Instagram says it heals all forms of illnesses, then you might want to think again.

In this book, I have not only presented my experiences drinking celery juice for more than two months, a decision I clearly regret, but I have also dug deep to find out if there are really existing studies to back the claims that celery is a be-all do-all miracle juice.

When I mean studies, I am talking about independent studies and scientific research, not something that someone whips up from "only God knows where" and claims it was revealed to them by "spirits."

Now, without further ado, let me show you why celery juice may not help you – this way, you do not raise your hopes unnecessarily, and you don't also have to waste your money juicing celery. Most importantly, you don't have to jeopardize your health even further by drinking celery juice. Please put on your seat belt; let's rock this ride together!

CHAPTER ONE

But celery is not new

The origin of celery cannot be easily traced; the reason is that there had never been a reason for scientists and researchers to carry out significant works about the plant. It was only recently that the plant started generating many buzzes that some scientists began to conduct some research on its origin. However, some ancient literature had traced the origin of celery to the Mediterranean basin.

Many ancient literature pieces contain records that lend credence to the assumption that as far as 850 B.C, celery and some other similar plants sharing the same family were cultivated and harvested for their medicinal properties. Many of the books documented that celery was used to relieve the effects of nerve pain, promote restful sleep, and control hysteria.

In the olden days, most jobs or activities were carried out manually. Hence, the people that lived in those days needed a lot of herbs to soothe their nerves and feel better after the typical day's hustle and bustle. And it was recorded that celery and some other plants were used for this purpose. Remember, the claims that celery was used in the days of old to soothe nerve pain is nothing more than a claim that has not been independently verified.

Many other literature works also documented that during ancient times, Ayurvedic physicians used the oil extracted from celery to treat and manage conditions such as water retention, poor digestion, cold, liver ailments, spleen ailments, and numerous types of arthritis.

Again, some of these were mere claims and have not been authenticated; the only sure thing is that celery does have some medicinal values, just like most other plants out there.

Ancient Egyptians were one of the oldest civilizations to have used celery, but surprisingly, they did not use it for food or medicinal values; instead, they used it to decorate tombs. Egyptians were known to conduct elaborate burials and build magnificent tombs. Some monuments of their ancient pharaohs still serve as tourist destinations even up to this day. They accorded much respect to the dead just as they respected the living.

That being said, the reason why ancient Egyptians decorated tombs using celery cannot really be ascertained, but some sources claim that the woven wreaths of celery which were usually used to decorate tombs were meant to keep the dead active as they made the transition from the land of the living to that of the deceased. That practice was based on superstitious beliefs – somehow. The Egyptians believed that celery had medicinal benefits but that it was only useful to the dead to help them navigate through the land of the dead peacefully.

Besides ancient Egyptians, ancient Greeks also used celery, which they considered a holy plant. Usually, winners of the Nemean Games would wear celery wreaths around their necks, similar to how winners of the Olympic Games today wear bay leaves. The first Nemean Games was in 573, and it used to be conducted once every second year in the small city of Nemea, south of Greece, in the Peloponnese peninsula.

It is clear that most ancient civilizations that used celery utilized it for purposes other than food and medicine. Only a few ancient civilizations like the Romans valued and used celery for cooking. Before the Romans, people were using celery to decorate tombs and celebrate winners of Nemean games.

After the Romans, the French were another group that used celery as food around 1623. For about a century, the French and the other civilizations that adopted celery as food only used it to flavor food. Early varieties of the plant had some form of spice; this made it an excellent flavoring agent in foods.

By the late 17th century and early 18th century, there were beginning to be visible improvements in the stalks of wild celery – this made it possible for it to become ideal for use in salads.

Through several trials and errors, gardeners discovered that all they needed to do to reduce celery's pungency was to grow it in colder weather. After this discovery, people started to use celery more and more in salads. Most salads were incomplete without celery.

Towards the middle of the 18th century, people had started storing celery in cellars, and only the affluent people in Northern Europe, especially during the winter, used them. By the end of the century, more and more people had adopted celery as food. Despite its wide popularity in Europe, it was not until 1806 before it was introduced to America by the colonists.

Since the early 20th century, celery has gained popularity in different countries and regions. Some of the places where celery is used for its nutritional values include China, New Zealand, Algeria, India, the United Kingdom, Egypt, the United States, Sweden, and many other countries.

Every 100 grams (3.9 ounces) of celery contains 18 calories – this means you can ingest high amounts of the plant without introducing an insane number of calories into your body. This could be why those who are promoting celery as the alpha and omega plant have claimed that it helps individuals lose weight. Whether celery makes people lose weight or not is something we shall find out later. We only know that celery has a healthy dose of a few vitamins and minerals.

Since celery became famous as a significant food ingredient, people have been using it to prepare smoothies, salads, and different kinds of foods. It was not until recently that a lot of people started exaggerating the health benefits of the plant.

Yes, celery has some health benefits, just like most other plants out there, but when some individuals begin to tout it as the miracle plant that heals all illnesses, we need to be worried.

A famous author Anthony William has been at the forefront of those promoting celery juice as the be-all do-all. In 2015, he started writing several posts about the health benefits of celery juice, and he soon gathered many followers. Before long, his followers had begun posting testimonials on Instagram, claiming to have been healed of all kinds of illnesses after drinking celery juice.

Note: William is not touting celery itself as the miracle plant; rather, he promotes the juice gotten from the plant as the miracle medicine. Because of the many bogus claims that William makes, I decided to try celery juice and see how it could help me deal with the acid reflux problems I was having.

Well, my results were not like what the other followers of Anthony were posting. Could it be that I did something wrong or that some of William's followers were posting lies? We shall get to find out soon.

CHAPTER TWO

The claims

In this section, we shall present some of the claims that have been made by those who promote celery juice as the be-all do-all in the health and wellness world. At the forefront of those making these claims is Anthony William, a man who says he is a Medical Medium (we shall see what a medium means later).

Sometime in 2018, William wrote an article published on Goop (Goop is owned by Gwyneth Paltrow, who is also known for her many controversial claims).

In the article, William referred to celery juice as the cure-all beverage capable of healing almost every sickness known to man. Because William and his celery juice sermons were already generating a lot of waves, more and more people started to believe that they could indeed be healed of their autoimmune diseases if they simply stick a stalk of celery in a juicer and drink the juice.

On *September 28, 2018*, the American musician Pharrell Williams posted a picture of himself on Instagram holding a glass of smoothies and captioned it, *"green juice."* Even though he did not state categorically that the juice in the glass was celery juice, his followers simply jumped to a conclusion and started proclaiming that the reason for the singer's ever-youthful appearance was the celery juice he drinks.

Even though Pharrell's followers had no real proof that what he was holding in the photo was celery juice, they simply chose to believe what their mind made up, probably because of the growing popularity of Anthony William, the man who had been claiming that celery juice was capable of healing almost all sicknesses.

According to Anthony William, if you just juice some celery stalks and drink the beverage first thing in the morning, then you are sure to be healed of almost all kinds of diseases. The broad claims are that celery contains some special types of mineral salts or salt clusters that suffocate disease-causing viruses and bacteria and make you whole.

According to William, drinking 16 ounces of celery juice in the morning on an empty stomach can heal you from all types of illnesses ranging from high blood pressure to migraines to different types of chronic diseases like rheumatoid arthritis. What is surprising in all of these is that William says that he is not a medical doctor or a licensed healthcare provider. So, how does he come up with all these claims? Well, he does say he is a Medical Medium.

What is a medium?

The word "medium" is not one you hear all the time except perhaps you are watching one of those horror movies of the 1950s. However, it is a word that has a real definition.

A medium refers to someone who claims to listen to or speak with non-existent entities such as spirits. Usually, mediums claim that they are in contact with higher spirits that reveal otherwise hidden things to them. Does that sound ridiculous enough? It does sound silly, and that is what Anthony William claims to be – he communicates with higher spirits who reveal medical secrets ahead of his time to him.

The issue of mediums has been a topic of great debate for ages. It is a myth that humans could communicate with spirits. Whether spirits exist or not is not the major issue of concern here; what is quite debatable is the claim that some humans possess the unique ability to communicate with higher beings called spirits.

For many years, charlatans who claim to be mediums have tricked people into giving up their money. Typically, the mediums use a series of psychological tricks to make their victims believe that they indeed have personal communication with non-existent spirits.

Some mediums are sometimes truthful and honest upfront about their trade. These types of mediums often call themselves mentalists, and they all use the same mental and psychological tricks to lure their victims into parting with their money.

In the real sense, mentalists and mediums usually do not communicate with any spirit. What they do instead is to leverage the services of assistants who provide them with information. This way, the unsuspecting victim would believe or think that the medium or mentalist got information about them from mysterious places.

Many people find them (mediums and mentalists) fascinating because even though lies are their stock in trade, it actually takes a lot of skills and mastery to identify signs and cues that could be used to dig up small unreliable facts about an individual or situation that could appear to come from the spirit world or mysterious places.

Furthermore, many delusional mediums actually believe that they have some magic powers and could communicate with spirits. A power that, on closer examination, you will find out does not exist.

Anthony William falls within this category. William and his fellow mediums prey on needy and sick people's ignorance and desperation and claim to hear the solution to their problems from the spirit world.

I have interviewed many people who have had encounters with mediums, and I was able to find out that mediums typically use two methods to convince their subjects or rather victims to believe that the medium is indeed passing hitherto hidden information to them. The mediums usually use a method called "reading" to unravel their victims' problems.

One reading method which is popular among mediums is known as "cold reading." In cold reading, a medium simply asks you questions about yourself and your condition and makes the whole thing appear like there is a spirit somewhere passing down the questions they ask you to them.

Anthony William does this well – the screenshot below shows perfectly well that William is deep into cold reading.

I paid $500 to have a reading with Anthony. I felt completely scammed and naïve for thinking someone would be able to properly diagnosis me in 30 min. over the phone. I was told he would be able to tell you what you have right away, and for the first half of my session he kept asking me questions about all my symptoms. He tells everyone they have EBV, including myself. He even told me some of my heavy metals were high, and I got tested right after and they were all low. I also found out through tests right after that my ASO and Streptozyme titers were extremely high and was diagnosed with Rheumatic Fever. He never once mentioned that.

I was completely desperate and still am since I am still sick, however I've learned my lesson the hard way. I just feel like I should let other people know what happened to me so they can save their money. Being sick is expensive!

I think his book is good and I do agree with some of the ideas, however after being so sick, reading so many health books and researching the internet for almost 1 1/2 years, I've learned to take everything you read with a grain of salt.

666 people found this helpful

Typically, the medium asks you open-ended questions, intending to extract as much information as possible from you. All along, they will be disguising themselves and make it appear like the questions they are asking you are from spirits.

Because you are already desperate, you will not know that the information they will feed you back and claim it was from the spirits was actually some of the information you supplied to them yourself. The medium usually does all these to make you believe that they can genuinely communicate with spirit entities.

While most mentalists or mediums do "*cold reading*" for the mere fun of it, many others do it purely for profit, and these are the dangerous ones because they can say anything just to fleece you.

From the moment you get in contact with them, they start observing cues in your mode of communication and your general body language; next, they use the observed signals to narrow their questions – this makes you excited, and you think they just got some revelations from spirits.

If there are really mentalists or mediums who hear from the spirits, then they should use their skills to become one of those millionaire poker players. But as you know, that will never happen because they are nothing but con artists and charlatans who feed on the desperation of solution seekers.

The other method that mediums and mentalists use when trying to convince their subjects that they (mentalists) are getting information from the spirit world is called *"hot reading."* To do "*hot reading,*" the mentalist or medium works with another person who is the co-conspirator – this person uses various means to get real information about the subject or victim.

Cold reading requires some special skills, unlike hot reading, where the co-conspirator could simply get information and pass them onto the medium or mentalist. At the same time, the latter transmits the information to their subject in a way that appears like a spirit was revealing the information.

In today's world, something as simple as access to Google could reveal all the information that the co-conspirator can transmit to their partner, which they could use to deceive an undiscerning subject.

The United States National Academy of Science once released a report on the issue of parapsychological phenomenon. The report was drawn from research conducted for over 130 years.

The report's simple conclusion was that there was no form of scientific or evidential justification for the existence of a parapsychological phenomenon in any kind or nature.

We have had several instances where a former mentalist or magician came out to debunk some of the claims that humans could speak to spirits. **James Randi** was one of such former mentalists who later became a serious skeptic of occult and spiritualism.

To further prove his points that humans cannot speak to spirits, James put up a challenge; he was ready to give $1 million to anyone willing to provide verifiable evidence that psychics could actually read minds or establish communication with spirits without the use of tricks. Up to this day, no one has taken up the challenge, which goes to show that all mediums and mentalists are con artists or charlatans.

If you dig a little deeper, you will find numerous stories where real skeptics have debunked hustlers who sell themselves as mediums with the ability to hear from spirits. By the time you remove tricks, you realize they possess no special powers like they often claim.

Having debunked the claims that mediums or mentalists communicate with higher beings, let's get to Medical Medium and some of his claims – that will be in the next chapter.

CHAPTER THREE

Medical Medium

Anthony William claims to be a Medical Medium who receives a diagnosis for all forms of sicknesses from spirits; he also makes a lot of bogus claims, including saying that celery juice is a heal-all beverage.

In the previous section, we saw that no evidence proves that humans or even psychics could speak with spirit beings. Now, one question you might want to ask yourself is, "*is Medical Medium any different from the other mediums or mentalists?*"

The bold answer is NO – Medical Medium is just like the other mediums who capitalize on the desperation of solution seekers. However, if you are not inclined to believing anecdotes as a real fact, or if you do not derive pleasure in believing carefully crafted new age fantasyland bullshit or pseudoscience, then you will definitely find it hard to see any unbiased evidence that Anthony William heals or even diagnoses any sickness correctly.

William said it himself that he is not a licensed medical practitioner, so he has no license to diagnose illnesses. Even the pseudoscience (e.g., naturopathy, chiropractic, etc.), which he parades himself as a master in, he has no real credentials in any of them.

If you independently verify and trace most of the people who claim to have been healed by him, you will find out that no real healing took place. This is something I have done myself – I monitored some of the people who claimed he healed them, and all of them are still suffering from their symptoms at the time of writing this book.

Unlike Medical Medium, a real physician does not rely on spirits to know the causes of illnesses and what solutions to offer. Through casual conversations and careful observations & laboratory tests, a certified and licensed healthcare provider will diagnose many severe conditions such as infections, neurological disorders, cancers, and other extreme health conditions.

To an accredited health practitioner, a cough could just mean that you have a cough, and it could also mean that you have an allergy, an infection, or a sign of a more serious condition like cancer. But to a medical medium; well, a cough could mean something deeper, and you may need the spirits' help to get better.

It could be that Medical Medium, just like a real healthcare provider, does have some observatory skills or an excellent psychological gift which he could use to deduce the cause of some minor health conditions.

One sure thing is: he cannot be trusted to diagnose dangerous health conditions like cancer and autoimmune diseases. He simply does not possess the qualification to diagnose such serious conditions (he admitted that he is not a doctor), except if all it takes to diagnose diseases these days is to watch 15 seasons of E.R on TV, then you may want to trust your health in the hands of someone who gets diagnoses from the spirit of "compassion."

Here is what Medical Medium claims about his powers:

Anthony William was born with the unique ability to converse with a high-level spirit who provides him with extraordinarily accurate health information that's often far ahead of its time. When Anthony was four years old, he shocked his family by announcing at the dinner table that his symptom-free grandmother had lung cancer. Medical testing soon confirmed the diagnosis.

For over 25 years, Anthony has devoted his life to helping people overcome and prevent illness—and discover the lives they were meant to live. What he does is several decades ahead of scientific discovery. His compassionate approach, which takes into account well-being on every level, not just physical health, has time and again given relief and results to those who seek him out.

Anthony's unprecedented accuracy and success rate as the Medical Medium have earned him the trust and love of thousands worldwide, among them movie stars, rock stars, billionaires, professional athletes, best-selling authors, and countless other people from all walks of life who couldn't find a way to heal until he provided them with insights from Spirit.

Unfortunately, I was part of those who blindly believed Medical Medium and took his recommendation that celery juice was a miracle juice seriously. Did I pay for it? Yes, I paid dearly for it; my health deteriorated to the extent that if I had not realized myself and stopped, it would have been late.

What if Medical Medium truly does hear from the spirits?

Okay, let's assume that Medical Medium does hear from the spirits; what advice do you think the spirit of "compassion" would typically give to this man? From his books, it seems the spirit of compassion convinced him that alternative medicine is the way out of all types of illness.

While I believe in alternative medicine, we cannot ignore the fact that what we know as alternative medicine is nothing more than everyday stuff we consume. For instance, Medical Medium talks so much about homeopathy; in fact, he is a big promoter of homeopathy. If you read his books, you understand that he promotes homeopathy a lot.

However, what is homeopathy? Is it not simply water therapy? And has it even been proven to be useful for the treatment of any illness? When you drink water, it helps to quench your thirst and keep you hydrated, and there is no evidence anywhere that proves that homeopathy, which is nothing more than water therapy, can treat any disease. But Medical Medium promotes homeopathy to be an ultimate healer.

Homeopathy is often referred to as the pseudoscience of water memory, and you could never find any physical, chemical, or biological law that backs water memory. If water memory is in any way plausible, don't you think the person who discovered it would be famous or renowned all over the world?

Yes, the person that discovered it would have been a renowned world figure, and we would have had to discard everything that science has taught us today and go the way of homeopathy.

The screenshot below shows Medical Medium prescribing homeopathy to one of his subjects.

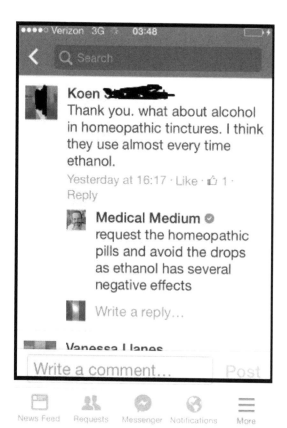

Bad advice

As stated earlier, it is surprising to discover that Medical Medium does not hold a license to practice in any field of medicine, but he somehow communicates with the spirits that tell him that solutions to almost any kind of disease are either celery juice, cucumbers, homeopathy, or other similar bullshit.

For instance, Medical Medium has on several occasions claimed that **artichokes** have unique abilities to stabilize or regulate blood sugar. Regulation of blood sugar is a critical issue for people suffering from diabetes, both type 1 and type 2.

While it is true that making the proper

food choices can help those living with diabetes to regulate or maintain a balanced blood glucose level; artichokes, however, cannot be trusted to do that alone.

The only thing that has been proven effective for the regulation of blood sugar levels in people with type 1 diabetes is the injection of insulin; artichokes do not even come close.

If someone with type 1 diabetes decides to eat artichokes all day, there will never be any difference in their health until they decide to do the right thing. Moreover, even if you decide to start eating artichokes, you cannot live on that alone; you still have to consider your overall diet and how they affect your blood sugar level if you have diabetes.

It is quite true that a variety of artichokes helps to regulate blood sugar levels; however, it is not the regular artichokes we eat; they are not even related. The artichokes in question here is called Jerusalem artichokes, which is not the type that William prescribes.

This type of artichokes helps to regulate blood sugar level due to the presence of a particular kind of glycoprotein which is usually found in its tuber. Jerusalem artichokes also helps to add fiber to the other foods you eat.

Unfortunately, Medical Medium promotes artichokes as one of the magical plants that heals all diseases. Once he has established through "reading" (which is just a fancy word for wild guessing) that his victim has diabetes, he goes ahead to ask the subject to start eating artichokes, an action that may further worsen the condition of the subject.

Cucumbers

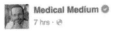

Medical Medium ✓
7 hrs · 🌐

Cucumbers are a highly alkalinizing and hydrating food that are rich in nutrients such as vitamins A, C, K, magnesium, silicon, and potassium. Cucumbers are also packed with antioxidants and enzymes such as erepsin which helps to digest proteins and destroy parasites and tapeworms.

The high chlorophyll and lignan content in the cucumber skin makes it a great anti-cancer food and can be particularly helpful in reducing the risk of estrogen related cancers such as breast, uterus, prostate, and ovarian cancer. The high fiber content of cucumbers makes it an excellent remedy for constipation by adding bulk and hydration directly to the colon.

Cucumbers are also one of the best natural diuretics around, aiding in the excretion of wastes through the kidneys and helping to dissolve uric acid accumulations such as kidney and bladder stones. They have wonderful anti-inflammatory benefits which can significantly benefit autoimmune and neurological disorders. It can also help to diminish swelling and puffiness underneath the eyes when applied externally.

Cucumbers also benefit teeth and gums as the fiber and nutrients help to massage the gums and remove bad bacteria from the teeth. Their high silica content promotes strong and healthy hair and nails which has earned them the reputation for centuries as being a "beautifying" food. Fresh cucumber juice has the ability to cleanse and detox the entire body as well as help to alleviate digestive problems such as gastritis, acidity, heartburn, indigestion, and ulcers.

It is also an ideal way to properly hydrate the body since it is contains beneficial electrolytes that have the ability to bring nutrients and hydration deep into the cells and tissues making it far more effective than water alone. Fresh cucumber juice is also an excellent remedy for bringing down a fever in children and the convalescent. 8-16oz fresh cucumber juice can rehydrate the body quickly and efficiently.

Learn more about which foods can heal and restore your body in my new book, click here http://bit.ly/mmbook02 ✪

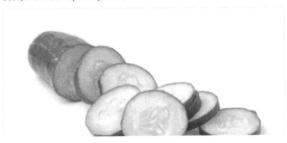

Apart from artichokes, Medical Medium also promotes cucumbers as the next superfood. Typically, Medical Medium would use his "magical abilities" to diagnose you with a long list of diseases, and next thing, he asks you to take cucumbers.

But aren't cucumbers just water? Cucumbers are just 95% water, and unlike what Medical Medium claims, cucumber is not truly rich in "special" nutrients. The only abundant nutrient in cucumber is vitamin K, which aids blood clotting.

Cucumbers do not contain erepsin, as opposed to claims by Medical Medium and other people like him. Erepsin is a member of a group of intestinal enzymes that aid digestion.

In the past, it was thought that cucumbers contained erepsin. Erepsin is not found in cucumbers; rather, they are produced by the intestinal tract. Also, erepsin does not destroy parasites in the stomach because, over the years, parasites in the gut have developed resistance to enzymes like erepsin and other similar ones.

Next, cucumbers are touted to be perfect diuretics. Again, cucumbers do not contain any diuretic compounds – except for their 95% water content. Since the fruit mostly contains water, it is not unnatural for you to urinate more often when you eat it – it is just your body's osmoregulation ability trying to push out the excess water you have ingested when you eat the fruit. Hence, there are no special compounds in cucumbers that promote diuresis.

Also, cucumber is not high in fiber, contrary to what most people think. The fiber content of cucumber is just as little as 1g of fiber for each large cucumber you eat. Eating a slice of wheat bread will give you more fiber (up to 5X more fiber) than consuming a big cucumber.

The almighty celery juice

Celery is currently one of the acclaimed superfoods being promoted by Medical Medium to be an ultimate healer. Apart from my own experience, which proved to me that celery is nothing more than a good plant that is being promoted for the wrong reasons, many other people have confirmed that celery juice does not perform all the wonders it is purported to perform.

In his usual manner, Medical Medium started promoting celery juice and even got celebrities to talk about taking celery juice first thing in the morning on an empty stomach.

Because many celebrities (including the most controversial ones like Kim Kardashian and Gwyneth Paltrow) talked about taking the juice after Medical Medium had hyped the beverage, the whole internet soon became agog, and a "#celeryjuicechallenge" was even started where people would take celery juice on an empty stomach for a week and claim to have been healed of all types of illnesses, then post their results on Instagram.

Medical Medium and many of the people who take celery juice claim that the juice helps people lose weight, get rid of acne, eczema, detoxify the liver, and improve gut health. Well, there is no real science anywhere that proves that celery juice can do any of these things. Celery juice does not contain any special compound (s) that detoxify the body except the "special salt clusters," which Medical Medium claims to have discovered in it.

Over time, real science has made us know that those claims about celery juice detoxifying the liver are nothing more than bare-faced lies that must be discarded. Neither celery juice nor any other fruit at all can detoxify the liver or the body.

This may come as a rude shock to you, but then, that's what it is. The liver and kidney are the organs with the primary responsibility of detoxifying the body. These organs have been made to perform their jobs perfectly whether you drink celery juice or not.

If you are already in the habit of eating many fruits every day and drinking a lot of water, then drinking celery juice will not do anything special to your body. The reason is simple; if you have been drinking a lot of water and eating many fruits, it means your body is already getting a healthy dose of vitamins and nutrients.

Now, if you start drinking celery juice, there is no other special nutrient or vitamin that celery juice will introduce to your body that you are not already getting. However, celery juice may help you get some vital nutrients and keep you hydrated if you have not been drinking much water and eating a lot of fruits.

Celery juice does not contain any special vitamin, nutrient, or "salt clusters" that are not found in other fruits. Celery contains vitamins C and K in healthy amounts. It also contains potassium and has a lot of water (a stalk of celery is about 95% water). All these mentioned nutrients and water in celery are not unique and are not different from the ones you find in other fruits.

So, if you already drink a lot of water and eat plenty of fruits that contain the same types of vitamins and minerals as celery, then you must not waste your money on celery juice.

You may want to ask, *"If drinking celery juice does not have any special effect, why is it that those that drank it had their acne cleared?"*

The answer is: hydration is vital for healthy-looking skin, and if you drink water more often, you will most likely have healthy-looking skin, free from acne and some other skin imperfections. Remember, celery has 95% water content, so when you drink it, you are introducing enough water into your body system, which may aid hydration.

Drinking celery juice will not make you more hydrated than drinking a few cups of water. So, if you could become consistent in drinking an amount of water equal in volume to 16 ounces of celery juice every day, then you will have clear skin too.

Furthermore, if you start drinking any other type of green juice today to increase the number of vitamins getting into your body and reduce the amount of sugars you consume, you will have good-looking skin as well.

As I have been reiterating, if you are already eating a well-balanced diet, drinking plenty of water, and having the right amount of fruits daily, then you will definitely not feel any different if you start consuming celery juice every morning on an empty stomach.

If you don't already drink a lot of water, eat lots of fruits, then you are better off skipping celery juice and start eating plenty of fruits as well as drinking a lot of water.

The claims by Medical Medium and other proponents of celery juice that it improves digestive health are totally false and cannot be substantiated. First, dietary fiber is one of the nutrients vital for a healthy gut.

When you eat fiber, it helps your bowels to move more regularly, aiding proper digestion. Fiber also keeps you full for a more extended period, and this may help you to consume fewer calories and consequently lose weight.

However, when you juice celery, you are getting rid of its fiber content, which is essentially what is right for gut health. You are only left with the juice, so if anyone tells you that drinking celery juice will improve your gut health, the person is a liar, and there is no truth in them.

Yes, eating celery as a whole without juicing may help your gut. Also, drinking celery smoothie, which contains fiber, may improve your gut health. Eating actual fruits and vegetables will improve your gut health. What will not improve your gut health is drinking celery juice because the fiber has been lost.

You might say, "but the juice contains a lot of vitamins, aren't those helpful?" Well, drinking celery juice may be more nutritious than drinking plain water because of the other vitamins and minerals found in celery juice which water does not have.

However, as mentioned earlier, if you are already getting those other minerals and vitamins from actual fruits and veggies, then drinking celery juice will not in any way do anything else special for you. You can take this to the bank!

Next, let's talk about the financial implication of juicing celery every morning – did you know that if you are just consuming celery as a snack, you will spend far less money than you would spend if you have to juice and drink it every morning?

This is not to mention the fact that the cost of a stalk of celery has almost doubled in the last couple of months, simply because a group of people listened to a man who gets instructions from spirits and started juicing celery every morning.

No evidence

There is no substantial evidence that any of the fruits that Medical Medium often prescribes as a cure for various illnesses works. Let's assume that we have chosen to give him (Medical Medium) the benefit of the doubt, and let's assume that he truly hears from spirits. Most of the treatment plans he would proffer to you will not work, and this I have shown in previous sections of this guide.

There is no evidence anywhere that drinking celery juice on an empty stomach first thing in the morning helps to clear the skin, especially for someone who already takes enough fruits and water daily.

There is no evidence that taking celery juice helps to improve gut health. But there is evidence that ignoring your medications and choosing to drink only celery juice because a medium (someone who hears from spirits) told you to do so can actually harm you. I shall talk more about this later.

There is also no available scientific evidence that artichokes, especially the common one we eat, helps regulate blood sugar levels. The only type of artichokes that remotely has anything to do with regulating blood sugar levels is Jerusalem artichokes, and surprisingly, Medical Medium does not even promote this type of artichokes.

There is no evidence that cucumbers help treat the myriads of health conditions that Medical Medium claims. Sadly, Medical Medium makes claims about severe health conditions like thyroid diseases, chronic fatigue syndrome, and autoimmune diseases, which all need a serious treatment plan handled by a trained health practitioner.

Then he (Medical Medium) claims that fruits (with no more than a few vitamins and minerals and much water) can heal those illnesses. It is even more absurd that he claims that he has the knowledge, some of which medical science will not know even in the next twenty years, and this supposedly special knowledge was revealed to him by spirits. I wonder what could be more absurd.

Yes, I was foolish enough to believe some of his claims at first, but have I learned my lessons? The answer is capital YES. However, what about the millions of people who believe in a man who claims to listen to spirits to treat a real serious mental health issue? More than once, he has said that he is not a trained healthcare provider. If you visit his

Facebook page, you will be able to download a PDF file containing a lengthy disclaimer which he uses to absolve himself of any blame should anything happen to his subjects. Here is just an excerpt from his disclaimer:

Anthony William, Inc. dba Anthony William, Medical Medium ("Anthony William, Medical Medium") is not a licensed medical doctor, chiropractor, osteopathic physician, naturopathic doctor, nutritionist, pharmacist, psychologist, psychotherapist, or other formally licensed healthcare professional, practitioner or provider of any kind. Anthony William, Medical Medium does not render medical, psychological, or other professional advice or treatment, nor does it provide or prescribe any medical diagnosis, treatment, medication, or remedy.

The information provided on and accessible from this page/website is for informational purposes only and should not be considered to be healthcare advice or medical diagnosis, treatment or prescribing. None of this information should be considered a promise of benefits, a claim of cures, a legal warranty or a guarantee of results to be achieved. This information is not intended as a substitute for advice from your physician or other healthcare professionals, or any notifications or instructions contained in or on any product label or packaging. You should not use this information for diagnosis or treatment of any health problem or for prescription of any medication or other treatment. You should consult with a healthcare professional before altering or discontinuing any current medications, treatment or care, starting any diet, exercise or supplementation program, or if you have or suspect you might have a health problem.

You can visit Medical Medium's Facebook page or website and view the full disclaimer. Here is a summary of the full disclaimer:

• Medical Medium (Anthony William) is not trained in any field of medicine (not even junk medicine like chiropractic or naturopathy), neither does he have the credentials to diagnose illnesses.

• The FDA has not been provided with any data; neither has it reviewed any data that proves that Medical Medium can accurately diagnose illnesses or treat those illnesses.

• Medical Medium is saying that he does not intend to diagnose a sickness nor proffer a solution, but that is precisely what he does. He then goes ahead to ask his subjects not to take his diagnoses and treatments as a substitute for scientific-based medicine.

• No one with biomedical background has

vetted Medical Medium's medical information.

Bottom line: Anthony William, Medical Medium, the man who started the whole celery juice craze, is not a trained medical doctor, neither does he have any license to practice in any field of medicine, not even chiropractic or naturopathy. He only uses the pseudoscience of "spiritual" readings (wild guesses) and alternative medicine to attempt to diagnose sicknesses and treat patients.

I was one of those who believed his many bogus claims about the superpowers of celery juice. In the next section, you will read about what happened to me when I drank celery juice for two months. Continue reading.

Let me hear your thoughts and comments about this book. Leave a review on the Amazon sales page of this book.

Other books by the same author:

1. <u>Inversion Therapy for Neck and Back Pain: How to Use the Inversion Table Therapy to Manage Neck Pain, Back Pain, and Sciatica</u>

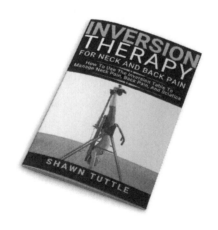

CHAPTER FOUR

Two months of drinking celery juice

Okay! So, after I heard about celery juice and how it was the miracle juice that cures all illnesses, I decided to incorporate it into my morning routine. For many years, I have been suffering from acid reflux, which happens to be one of the illnesses that Medical Medium claims that celery juice cures.

Before I started, I had read one of Medical Medium's books where he claimed that to get the best results from celery juice, one has to take it on an empty stomach first thing in the morning.

According to Medical Medium, when you juice the plant with other veggies or fruits, those fruits or vegetables will dilute and reduce celery's organic mineral content.

I had to wait till a particular Saturday to try celery juice because I was not sure of what to expect, so I wanted to make sure I took it on a day that I would not go out. That way, if my stomach started reacting to the juice, it would be that I was at home where I could easily take care of myself.

The previous day, being Friday, I had gone to the grocery store and bought some stalks of celery. Since I did not have a masticating juicer, I also got one because masticating juicers were the best for juicing celery.

On that fateful Saturday morning, I woke up around 6 AM. Without doing anything else, not even brushing my teeth, I dashed to my kitchen, grabbed one stalk of celery, fixed my new juicer, and within a few minutes, I had some celery juice collected in a glass. Since the juice from just one stalk was not up to the 16 ounces that Medical Medium recommends, I decided to juice one more stalk.

To be clear, I washed the plant in plenty of water before juicing. I also removed the root buds as well as the leaves. So, you cannot say that I did not prepare the juice properly. I had heard that juicing both the leaves of the plant makes the juice taste bitter, so I often removed the leaves because I wouldn't say I like awful tastes.

After the entire preparation, I was ready to drink my first glass of celery juice. I had read a lot about the omnipotence of celery, and I was really enthusiastic that the juice was going to work wonders in my body. Well, whether that happened or not is what you will find out soon.

Taste

I could not pinpoint what it tasted like on my first try. I would later learn that celery juice tastes differently to different people. That first time, it tasted like some salted grass to me. I have heard people say it tastes like a combination of salt and baking soda. I have also heard someone say it tastes like the outer skin of sugar cane.

The taste of your celery juice, as I heard, will depend on the parts of the plant you included in the juice.

Note: for the two months I tried celery juice, I used to cut out the leaves. You need to know that celery does not taste good, it has an awful taste, and it doesn't matter the part of the plant you added in the juice.

Side effects

Remember, you are told to drink celery juice in the morning before taking other foods, even water, and that was the instruction I followed. Medical Medium claims that taking celery juice this way will enable the *"nutrients and phytonutrients"* in the juice to find their way into your body system as fast as possible and start working wonders.

Now, one thing you will never hear elsewhere is that drinking celery juice comes with some unpleasant side effects. So, if you are drinking it to help you relieve the symptoms of any stomach-related health condition like IBS (irritable bowel syndrome), stomach acidity, then you may be in for an awful experience. Also, if you have low blood pressure, you may be subjecting yourself to more harm by drinking celery juice.

That being said, on the first day I took celery juice, I was enthusiastic that I was going to get healed miraculously. I do remember some things that did happen that day. It was on a Saturday, just like I stated earlier. So, I was not going out, and I used the opportunity to try out the juice.

I do remember that on that first day, after an hour or so, my stomach kind of started turning a little. I am not saying this would happen to you, but I experienced a mild stomach upset.

I thought that was happening because it was my first time trying the juice. However, when I had the same experience on the second day, I knew something was wrong.

Also, on that first day, I could not finish the entire 16 ounces I prepared because after I had gone halfway, I started feeling nauseous. This is me being honest; while I am not saying the juice will make you feel nauseous, I just want to share my experiences with you.

On the second day, being Sunday, I could remember that the juice did not taste better. One remarkable thing was that I took the entire 16 ounces I prepared on this second day, and after about two hours, I felt like throwing up, but the feeling was not as strong as what I felt on the first day.

On both the first and second day, I felt so bloated that it felt as if I was an inflated balloon. As someone that had suffered acid reflux for so long, I was already used to feeling bloated; however, celery juice made the bloating so scary.

It was a huge surprise to me since celery juice was being touted as a miracle juice that reduces bloating. It was also a surprise to me that celery juice was making me feel nauseous.

The feeling of nausea is one of the symptoms of acid reflux, and I was hoping drinking celery juice was going to, at least, reduce my symptoms, but it increased it, instead.

I may not be able to document my daily experiences here for the two months I took celery juice, but one thing you would want to take away is that it never got better each day. Each day came with its own challenge.

I was holding on to the routine, thinking that maybe, tomorrow, I could find the relief I was desperately seeking. However, it never came, and after two painful months, I had to stop.

Note: before I started taking celery juice, I took proton pump inhibitors (these are meant to inhibit the production of excess acid in the stomach). Usually, I would take the drugs for 14 days at a stretch, then take a break and resume retaking the pills.

I was doing it that way because taking proton pump inhibitors for an extended period could lead to osteoporosis. When I started taking celery juice, I could not take the proton pump inhibitors for two straight months, and the consequences of that action were dire. When I eventually stopped drinking celery juice totally, I had jeopardized my health greatly, that I had to be admitted to the hospital.

Apart from not being able to heal me of acid reflux, drinking celery juice for two months did not significantly change my skin tone. Okay, I am a man; I am not supposed to be bothered about my skin tone.

Yes, I am not bothered about that, but those touting celery juice as the alpha and omega said it could help you get smooth flawless skin. Typically, I was hoping that since drinking the juice could not help with my acid reflux condition, at least, it should help make me an ageless man. However, did that happen? The answer is capital NO.

As mentioned earlier, it is only those who have not been drinking a lot of water and eating plenty of fruits before drinking celery juice that may see anything that remotely resembles an improvement in their skin tone.

If you already have a habit of drinking plenty of water, which helps your skin and other organs to be well hydrated, you will not see any difference if you start drinking celery juice. I mentioned earlier that my daughter drank celery juice too, and it did not make any difference in the acne on her face.

One big lie

One big lie you might have heard is that when you experience side effects, it is a sign that the celery juice is detoxifying your body. In the previous section, you saw that the only organs in your body responsible for getting toxins out of your body are your liver and kidney, and drinking celery juice will never make any difference.

Detoxification is another buzzword that people have used to create a multi-billion dollar industry. If you spend a few hours in the science section of any library, or if you do something as simple as an internet search, you will find well-researched books, properly documented and referenced journals, that all debunk the detoxification lie.

Celery juice will not detoxify your body. The symptoms you experience after drinking the juice indicate that it is causing damage to your body, and you must take precautions.

More typical side effects

One other symptom you might experience when you drink celery is diarrhea. While I did not have diarrhea when I was taking the juice, I remember that few people close to me had it when they took the juice. Again, they may tell you that diarrhea results from the celery juice detoxifying your body; that's a huge lie.

Celery juice worsens irritable bowel syndrome (IBS)

If you have IBS (Irritable Bowel Syndrome), then you must stay away from celery juice. FODMAP is a member of a group of compounds that are thought to contribute to irritable bowel syndrome symptoms, and surprisingly, celery juice contains FODMAP. If you react to FODMAP, consuming up to 16 ounces of celery juice will cause you to experience some symptoms.

There are many other adverse side effects of drinking celery juice, and I may not list all of them here. I spoke with a friend who had been battling with high blood pressure and type II diabetes. He told me that after taking celery juice, his blood pressure got raised even higher.

According to claims, celery juice was supposed to lower his blood pressure; however, my friend experienced the exact opposite.

WRAP UP

After reading the overwhelming evidence presented in this book which shows that celery juice is not the miracle beverage it was touted to be, would you still drink celery juice and hope it heals you of your diseases?

While there is nothing wrong with taking celery as a snack, you will only feel disappointed when you juice it and expect it to heal you of all your infirmities. I learned early in life that once a fruit, drug, or food is being touted as a be-all do-all, then in most cases, it does not always turn out well.

If you could just put on your thinking cap for a few minutes and go down memory lane, you would realize that most foods that have ever been proposed as an alpha and omega usually turn out to be just like other common foods with little or no extra medicinal value.

Was it not just some months back that CBD oil was being touted as the be-all do-all? Today, you cannot point to one person and say, "this person took CBD oil and was healed."

Please, do not misunderstand me; CBD oil has medicinal values, although that assertion is subject to debate as there is no science to back it up. However, what I strongly disagree with is that it heals all types of illnesses.

Now, you may ask, "Why do people who start these trends do so?" Nothing more than the urge to make quick profits. People like Medical Medium know that by telling you all the time that celery juice heals all kinds of sicknesses, you would be tempted to purchase his books and read more about celery.

It is never about you; it is always about them. Perhaps, after reading the things the "spirit of compassion" revealed to him, you might be tempted to call in for a "reading." We talked about cold and hot reading in a previous section of this guide. When you call in for a reading, he tells you some incoherent stuff and claims he had heard them from the spirits. Then you end up wasting both your money and time.

The thought that drinking celery juice in the morning on an empty stomach would cure one of any serious illnesses like thyroid disease is totally absurd. What even makes these claims more unreasonable is the fact that the person telling you to do it claims to have gotten such instructions from "spirits." If you want to understand how ridiculous that sounds, then imagine this scenario:

You just got on the plane, and the pilot announces that he is not a trained pilot, but he trusts spirits to guide him on how to pilot the aircraft and take you to your destination. Without wasting time, you would get down from the plane and find your way simply because you cannot entrust your precious life in the hands of "spirits."

How then are there people who are willing to entrust their life in the hands of someone who clearly states it that he is not a trained or licensed medical practitioner but a Medical Medium who gets diagnoses from spirits?

Truly, drinking celery juice may help you get good-looking skin, but that is only possible if you have not been drinking enough water and eating a lot of fruits earlier. If you have been doing all that, then drinking celery juice will not make any difference (not even the slightest difference) on your skin.

Also, if you are suffering from any serious health condition such as thyroid disease, autoimmune disorders, cancer, or any other serious illnesses that celery juice is claimed to cure, then you must never drink celery juice and hope it cures you.

Yes, if you like bitter-tasting juices, then there is no harm in drinking celery juice. If you like wasting your money, you may consider juicing celery and drinking every morning. However, if you aim to manage or treat a serious health condition, you must trust and seek a trained healthcare provider's advice over that of someone who claims to hear from spirits.

Thanks for reading this book to the end. Let me hear your thoughts and comments about what you just read. Leave a review on the Amazon sales page of this book.

Other books by the same author:

1. Inversion Therapy for Neck and Back Pain: How to Use the Inversion Table Therapy to Manage Neck Pain, Back Pain, and Sciatica

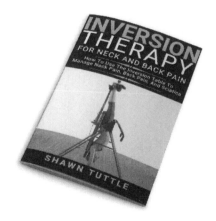

ABOUT THE AUTHOR

Shawn Tuttle is a writer, researcher, recipe developer, and music enthusiast. For more than two decades, he has developed and written tons of insightful texts on health and fitness related topics. Many professionals like chefs, fitness coaches, health, and food enthusiasts have found his books useful. When he is not researching and writing on exciting issues, he is trying to write HTML codes his for dog training website or making some nice tunes on his guitar.

DON'T Drink Celery Juice, Drink Water Instead

DON'T Drink Celery Juice, Drink Water Instead

DON'T Drink Celery Juice, Drink Water Instead